MAMA'S MILK & ME

MAMA'S MILK & ME

A Countdown Journal
for Nursing Mothers

By *Alisha Gaddis*

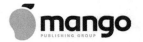

mango
PUBLISHING GROUP

CORAL GABLES

For permission requests, please contact the publisher at:
Mango Publishing Group
2850 S Douglas Road, 2nd Floor
Coral Gables, FL 33134 USA
info@mango.bz

For special orders, quantity sales, course adoptions and
corporate sales, please email the publisher at sales@mango.
bz. For trade and wholesale sales, please contact Ingram
Publisher Services at customer.service@ingramcontent.com or
+1.800.509.4887.

Mama's Milk and Me: A Countdown Journal for
Nursing Mothers

Library of Congress Cataloging-in-Publication number:
2020940936

ISBNs: (p) 978-1-64250-384-5 (e) 978-1-64250-385-2

BISAC: FAM032000, FAMILY & RELATIONSHIPS / Parenting /
Motherhood

Printed in the United States of America

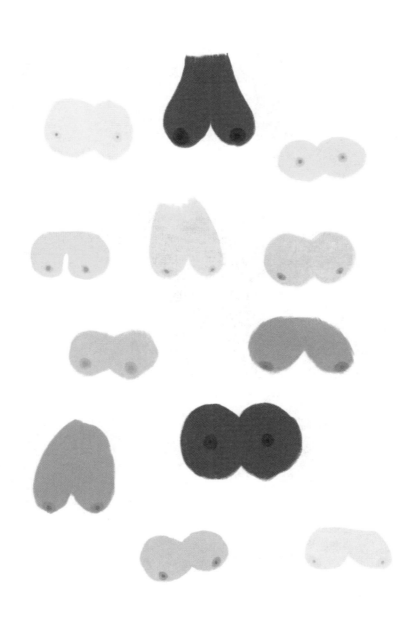

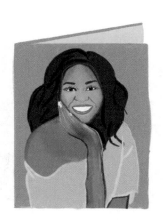

"Being a *Mother* has been a master class in letting go."

— *Michelle Obama*

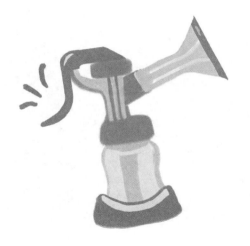

Note to Mothers from a Mother

You have been able to feed your child with your milk! What a fabulous gift to your most beloved! Whether it was difficult or easy, whether you supplemented or pumped, whether it was two weeks, two months, two years, or beyond—your time was special. Just you and your baby—early mornings, middle of the nights, roadsides, hotel rooms, beaches, and sun-filled porches.

Weaning is one of the hardest, most powerful, and most hormone-induced times of your life as a Mama. This new stage is just that—new. The emotional and physical bond between you and your child will continue to thrive and evolve as you grow together. Still, the separation is definitely difficult.

This book will help you both adapt.

Use it as a guide, tool, and keepsake. Fill in with your own story, your own experiences, and your own hopes!

I began sharing this dialogue with my daughter about two weeks before I nursed her for a final time. I began by repeating phrases such as, "Mama's Milk is only for you, but it has done its job and it will be gone soon." "I love you, always." "You are such a big, strong person!" Etc.

She would always listen and cuddle in closer.

As the time grew near, we read more and talked about funny nursing experiences. (Rather, I was talking, while she was slurping up my perfect drink made especially for her.) I knew our time was coming to an end. I wanted to make it last even longer and remember it all. It really does go by so very quickly!

We began the countdown of seven days to a "Bye Bye Mama's Milk Party" a.k.a. "I Am a Big Kid Party" that included a long, last nursing session. I can still remember how the light streamed in from the curtains. I wept and she held on tightly for what seemed like days. After she finished, I dried my tears and we put on fancy dresses (she was 23.5 months). We ate cupcakes and had a pizza party with daddy. Then we went to her favorite kids' museum and had the most special day. Almost like a birthday! And if you think about it, it is the birth of a new chapter.

I fully believe all of this helped ease both of us into this transition and new terrain.

I hope this book helps you celebrate and remember. Please use it just like that. With ease, joy, and truth.

Much love,
Alisha

Weaning can cause hormonal challenges for women, so check in with your care provider as you begin and after for support. Please show yourself care. You deserve it.

What adventures we have together,

_____
(child's name) & Mama!

What special times.

So far, Mama has been able to give you her milk to make you big, strong, smart, and brave in this world. Mama's Milk was made only for you.

Just like us—it was meant to be.

But Mama's Milk is almost done. You are big and strong and no longer need it to grow.

I remember when you were born and were a tiny, little baby. You were so hungry. You took to mama's

breast to drink _____
(quickly, easily, with difficulty, etc.).

In your own way.

That was just the beginning!

Every day, you needed more and more of Mama's Milk to grow and grow! Sometimes, I nursed you

_____ times a day!

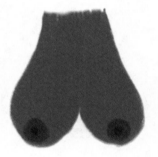

" Human milk is like ice cream, penicillin, and the drug ecstasy wrapped up in two pretty packages."

—Florence Williams

I REMEMBER ONCE YOU HAD MAMA'S MILK IN

(THE SILLIEST PLACE YOU EVER NURSED).

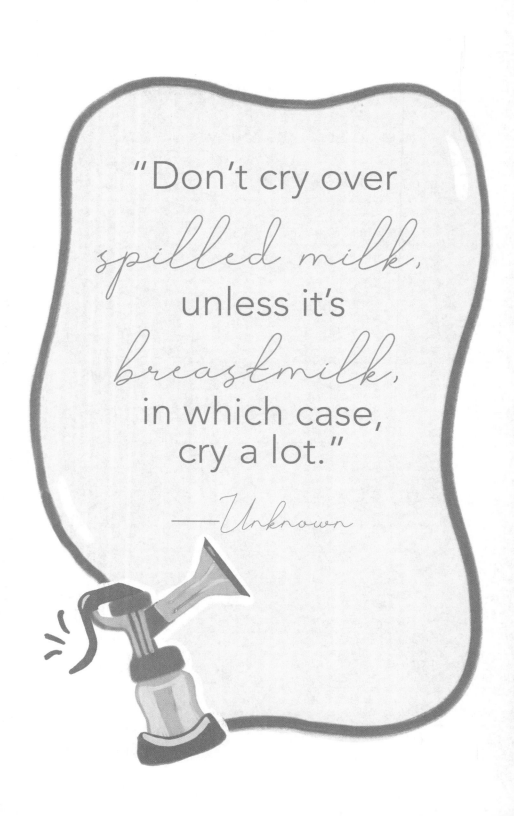

"Don't cry over spilled milk, unless it's breastmilk, in which case, cry a lot."

—Unknown

YOU ALWAYS LOVED TO NURSE RIGHT WHEN

_____

_____

(you got up from a nap, it was bedtime, before
bath, etc.).

_____

_____

_____

_____

_____

_____

_____

_____

_____

_____

_____

_____

_____

MAMA'S MILK WAS MADE JUST FOR YOU!

"The days are
long, but the years
are short."

—Gretchen Rubin

I NEVER WANT TO FORGET MY SWEETEST
MEMORY OF NURSING, WHICH WAS

_____

_____

_____

_____

_____

_____

_____

_____

_____

_____

_____

_____

_____

_____

_____

_____

_____

_____

_____

TAKE A MOMENT OF STILLNESS.
BREATHE IN YOU AND YOUR BABY.

**SOMETIMES, YOU WOULD FALL ASLEEP
IN MY ARMS WHEN I WAS NURSING YOU.
YOUR FACE LOOKED JUST LIKE**

_____

_____

_____

_____

_____

_____

_____

_____

_____

_____

_____

_____

_____

_____

_____

_____

_____

_____

_____

_____

Your favorite distractions while nursing:

- ♥ _____
- ♥ _____
- ♥ _____
- ♥ _____
- ♥ _____
- ♥ _____
- ♥ _____
- ♥ _____
- ♥ _____

Mine:

- ♥ _____
- ♥ _____
- ♥ _____
- ♥ _____
- ♥ _____
- ♥ _____
- ♥ _____
- ♥ _____
- ♥ _____

I WAS GIVEN/BOUGHT THIS SILLY THING FOR YOU THAT I THOUGHT I NEEDED, BUT I DON'T:

_____

_____

_____

_____

_____

_____

_____

_____

_____

_____

_____

_____

_____

_____

_____

_____

_____

_____

"A newborn baby has only three demands. They are

1. Warmth in the arms of its mother

2. Food from your breasts

3. Security in the knowledge of her presence

Breastfeeding satisfies all three."

—Grandly Dick-Reed

WHEN I'M GIVING YOU MAMA'S MILK, SOMETIMES MY MIND WANDERS.

I think about:

_____

_____

_____

_____

_____

_____

_____

I dream about:

_____

_____

_____

_____

_____

_____

_____

I worry about:

_____
_____
_____
_____
_____
_____
_____
_____
_____
_____

I wish:

_____
_____
_____
_____
_____
_____
_____
_____
_____
_____
_____

I HAVE SO MANY PLANS FOR US!
SOMEDAY I WANT TO TAKE YOU TO:

♥ _____

♥ _____

♥ _____

♥ _____

♥ _____

_____

_____

_____

_____

_____

_____

_____

_____

_____

_____

_____

_____

_____

_____

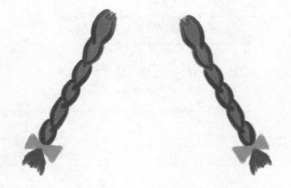

"I feel like a milkmaid, but it's worth it."

— *Miranda Kerr*

WHEN YOU ARE NURSING, SOMETIMES I LOOK AT YOUR FACE AND WONDER WHAT YOU ARE THINKING ABOUT.

Maybe

or

Could it be...

or

"Scared, afraid, sad, proud. Honor all your feelings as you both wean."

—Alisha Gaddis

Sometimes, it is lonely nursing, but sometimes I feel more full of love than I have ever felt. This is something I want you to know as you go through this world. Even if you feel lonely, you are never alone. I am right here with you.

Ways I give you care other than nursing you:

-
-
-
-
-

_____

_____

_____

_____

_____

_____

_____

_____

_____

_____

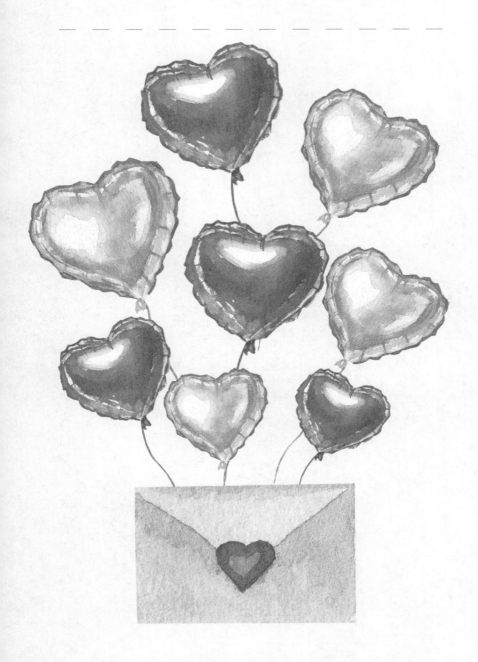

THE NAMES IN THESE HEARTS ARE JUST SOME
OF THE PEOPLE THAT LOVE YOU, MY BABY.

"Nursing gives
you superpowers."

—Gwen Stefani

YOUR FIRST FOODS ARE/OR WILL BE

_____

_____

_____

_____

_____

_____

_____

_____

_____

_____

_____

_____

I'VE DRAWN THEM HERE:

"All children
wean eventually."

—Unknown

SO MANY MILESTONES ARE HAPPENING IN YOUR LIFE OUTSIDE OF NURSING, LIKE

YOU ARE CHANGING SO MUCH PHYSICALLY.
HERE IS WHAT I HAVE NOTICED, MY LOVE.

"We all have nipples.
I don't care who I
offend. My baby
wants to eat."

—Selma Blair

I FEEL SO MANY EMOTIONS WHEN
I AM WEANING YOU. LIKE:

_____

_____

_____

_____

_____

_____

_____

_____

_____

_____

_____

_____

_____

_____

_____

_____

_____

_____

"I make milk. What is your superpower?"

—Unknown

Here is what I am doing:

_____
_____
_____
_____
_____
_____
_____
_____
_____

Watching:

_____
_____
_____
_____
_____
_____
_____
_____
_____
_____

Reading:

Listening to:

While I nurse you.

HERE ARE SOME THINGS TO BE HAPPY ABOUT.

"Little children, from
the moment they
are weaned, are
making their way
toward independence."

—Maria Montessori

THERE ARE SO MANY OTHER WAYS YOU AND I ARE CLOSE. HERE ARE SOME OF THEM:

_____

_____

_____

_____

_____

_____

_____

_____

_____

_____

_____

_____

_____

_____

_____

_____

_____

_____

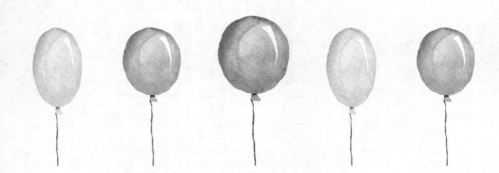

"I had given him so much throughout our time breastfeeding, and how it ended wouldn't and didn't take anything away from that."

—Allyson Lux

HERE IS A TYPICAL DAY IN OUR
LIVES TOGETHER:

Wake-up:

_____

_____

_____

_____

_____

_____

Mid-day:

_____

_____

_____

_____

_____

Afternoon:

_____

_____

_____

_____

_____

_____

Evening:

_____
_____
_____
_____
_____
_____

Nighttime:

_____
_____
_____
_____
_____
_____
_____
_____

Late Night:

_____
_____
_____
_____
_____
_____

"Every natural
weaning is unique,
so it is impossible to
guarantee anything
about it, except that
it will happen."

— Norma Jean
Bumgarner,
Mothering your Nursing Toddler

"It is ok to mourn the end of nursing your child."

—Alisha Gaddis

I AM SO PROUD OF YOU,

_____

(child's name)

_____
_____
_____
_____
_____
_____
_____
_____
_____
_____
_____
_____
_____
_____
_____
_____
_____
_____
_____

Coming to the End of Nursing

Feel free to read this to your baby every day,
evolving it as you see fit. Remember, this is YOUR
journey. There is no right way. There is no success,
there is no failure. You are enough.

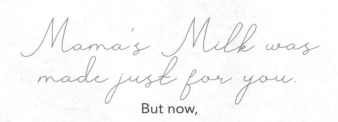

Mama's Milk was made just for you.
But now,

_____
(name of child),
you are big and strong. Mama's Milk has done its
job, and soon it will be gone. You don't need it
anymore. You will continue to grow and grow!

You are ready for this.
You are ready to be in the world and have

_____
(cow's milk, almond milk, juice, etc.).

But do not fret, you and mama will always be
together and have adventures! In my heart, you will
always be mama's baby.

We are going to count down to the end of Mama's
Milk together.

MAMA'S MILK WILL BE GONE ON _____.

THAT'S IN _____ **DAYS.**

We are going to celebrate it in the biggest way!
We are going to:

_____

_____

_____

_____

It will be a party to thank Mama's Milk and to
CELEBRATE you growing up big and strong!

**I AM SO PROUD OF YOU AND I AM SO PROUD
OF ME. WE DID THIS TOGETHER.**

_____

_____

_____

_____

_____

_____

_____

_____

_____

_____

_____

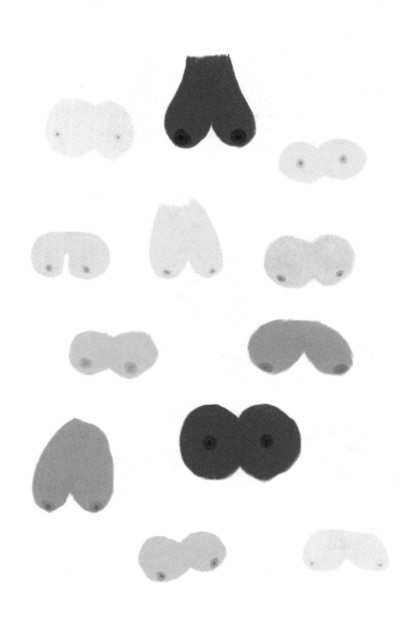

THE END
OF NURSING
COUNTDOWN

_____ MONDAY

GOAL:

_____

HOW I'M FEELING:

_____

HOW THE BABY IS DOING:

_____

WHAT ELSE IS GOING ON:

_____

_____ TUESDAY

GOAL:

_____

HOW I'M FEELING:

_____

HOW THE BABY IS DOING:

_____

WHAT ELSE IS GOING ON:

_____

_____ WEDNESDAY

GOAL:

_____

HOW I'M FEELING:

_____

HOW THE BABY IS DOING:

_____

WHAT ELSE IS GOING ON:

_____

_____ THURSDAY

GOAL: _____

HOW I'M FEELING: _____
_____

HOW THE BABY IS DOING: _____
_____

WHAT ELSE IS GOING ON: _____

_____ FRIDAY

GOAL: _____

HOW I'M FEELING: _____
_____

HOW THE BABY IS DOING: _____
_____

WHAT ELSE IS GOING ON: _____

_____ SATURDAY

_____ SUNDAY

_____ MONDAY

GOAL: _____

HOW I'M FEELING: _____

HOW THE BABY IS DOING: _____

WHAT ELSE IS GOING ON: _____

_____ TUESDAY

GOAL: _____

HOW I'M FEELING: _____

HOW THE BABY IS DOING: _____

WHAT ELSE IS GOING ON: _____

_____ WEDNESDAY

GOAL: _____

HOW I'M FEELING: _____

HOW THE BABY IS DOING: _____

WHAT ELSE IS GOING ON: _____

_____THURSDAY

GOAL: _____

_____
HOW I'M FEELING: _____

_____
HOW THE BABY IS DOING: _____

_____
WHAT ELSE IS GOING ON: _____

_____ FRIDAY

GOAL: _____

_____
HOW I'M FEELING: _____

_____
HOW THE BABY IS DOING: _____

_____
WHAT ELSE IS GOING ON: _____

_____ SATURDAY

_____ SUNDAY

_____ MONDAY

GOAL:

HOW I'M FEELING:

HOW THE BABY IS DOING:

WHAT ELSE IS GOING ON:

_____ TUESDAY

GOAL:

HOW I'M FEELING:

HOW THE BABY IS DOING:

WHAT ELSE IS GOING ON:

_____ WEDNESDAY

GOAL:

HOW I'M FEELING:

HOW THE BABY IS DOING:

WHAT ELSE IS GOING ON:

_____ THURSDAY

GOAL:

HOW I'M FEELING:

HOW THE BABY IS DOING:

WHAT ELSE IS GOING ON:

_____ FRIDAY

GOAL:

HOW I'M FEELING:

HOW THE BABY IS DOING:

WHAT ELSE IS GOING ON:

_____ SATURDAY

_____ SUNDAY

_____ MONDAY

GOAL:

_____

_____

HOW I'M FEELING:

_____

_____

HOW THE BABY IS DOING:

_____

_____

WHAT ELSE IS GOING ON:

_____

_____

_____ TUESDAY

GOAL:

_____

_____

HOW I'M FEELING:

_____

_____

HOW THE BABY IS DOING:

_____

_____

WHAT ELSE IS GOING ON:

_____

_____

_____ WEDNESDAY

GOAL:

_____

_____

HOW I'M FEELING:

_____

_____

HOW THE BABY IS DOING:

_____

_____

WHAT ELSE IS GOING ON:

_____

_____

_____ THURSDAY

GOAL: _____

_____

HOW I'M FEELING: _____

_____

HOW THE BABY IS DOING: _____

_____

WHAT ELSE IS GOING ON: _____

_____ FRIDAY

GOAL: _____

_____

HOW I'M FEELING: _____

_____

HOW THE BABY IS DOING: _____

_____

WHAT ELSE IS GOING ON: _____

_____ SATURDAY

_____ SUNDAY

_____ MONDAY

GOAL:

HOW I'M FEELING:

HOW THE BABY IS DOING:

WHAT ELSE IS GOING ON:

_____ TUESDAY

GOAL:

HOW I'M FEELING:

HOW THE BABY IS DOING:

WHAT ELSE IS GOING ON:

_____ WEDNESDAY

GOAL:

HOW I'M FEELING:

HOW THE BABY IS DOING:

WHAT ELSE IS GOING ON:

_____ THURSDAY

GOAL: _____

_____

HOW I'M FEELING: _____

_____

HOW THE BABY IS DOING: _____

_____

WHAT ELSE IS GOING ON: _____

_____ FRIDAY

GOAL: _____

_____

HOW I'M FEELING: _____

_____

HOW THE BABY IS DOING: _____

_____

WHAT ELSE IS GOING ON: _____

_____ SATURDAY

_____ SUNDAY

_____ MONDAY

GOAL:

HOW I'M FEELING:

HOW THE BABY IS DOING:

WHAT ELSE IS GOING ON:

_____ TUESDAY

GOAL:

HOW I'M FEELING:

HOW THE BABY IS DOING:

WHAT ELSE IS GOING ON:

_____ WEDNESDAY

GOAL:

HOW I'M FEELING:

HOW THE BABY IS DOING:

WHAT ELSE IS GOING ON:

_____THURSDAY

GOAL: _____

HOW I'M FEELING: _____

HOW THE BABY IS DOING: _____

WHAT ELSE IS GOING ON: _____

_____ FRIDAY

GOAL: _____

HOW I'M FEELING: _____

HOW THE BABY IS DOING: _____

WHAT ELSE IS GOING ON: _____

_____ SATURDAY

_____ SUNDAY

_____ MONDAY

GOAL:

HOW I'M FEELING:

HOW THE BABY IS DOING:

WHAT ELSE IS GOING ON:

_____ TUESDAY

GOAL:

HOW I'M FEELING:

HOW THE BABY IS DOING:

WHAT ELSE IS GOING ON:

_____ WEDNESDAY

GOAL:

HOW I'M FEELING:

HOW THE BABY IS DOING:

WHAT ELSE IS GOING ON:

_____ THURSDAY

GOAL:

HOW I'M FEELING:

HOW THE BABY IS DOING:

WHAT ELSE IS GOING ON:

_____ FRIDAY

GOAL:

HOW I'M FEELING:

HOW THE BABY IS DOING:

WHAT ELSE IS GOING ON:

_____ SATURDAY

_____ SUNDAY

_____ MONDAY

GOAL:

HOW I'M FEELING:

HOW THE BABY IS DOING:

WHAT ELSE IS GOING ON:

_____ TUESDAY

GOAL:

HOW I'M FEELING:

HOW THE BABY IS DOING:

WHAT ELSE IS GOING ON:

_____ WEDNESDAY

GOAL:

HOW I'M FEELING:

HOW THE BABY IS DOING:

WHAT ELSE IS GOING ON:

_____ THURSDAY

GOAL: _____

_____

HOW I'M FEELING: _____

_____

HOW THE BABY IS DOING: _____

_____

WHAT ELSE IS GOING ON: _____

_____ FRIDAY

GOAL: _____

_____

HOW I'M FEELING: _____

_____

HOW THE BABY IS DOING: _____

_____

WHAT ELSE IS GOING ON: _____

_____ SATURDAY

_____ SUNDAY

_____ MONDAY

GOAL:

HOW I'M FEELING:

HOW THE BABY IS DOING:

WHAT ELSE IS GOING ON:

_____ TUESDAY

GOAL:

HOW I'M FEELING:

HOW THE BABY IS DOING:

WHAT ELSE IS GOING ON:

_____ WEDNESDAY

GOAL:

HOW I'M FEELING:

HOW THE BABY IS DOING:

WHAT ELSE IS GOING ON:

_____ THURSDAY

GOAL: _____

HOW I'M FEELING: _____

HOW THE BABY IS DOING: _____

WHAT ELSE IS GOING ON: _____

_____ FRIDAY

GOAL: _____

HOW I'M FEELING: _____

HOW THE BABY IS DOING: _____

WHAT ELSE IS GOING ON: _____

_____ SATURDAY

_____ SUNDAY

_____ MONDAY

GOAL:

_____

HOW I'M FEELING:

_____
_____

HOW THE BABY IS DOING:

_____
_____

WHAT ELSE IS GOING ON:

_____
_____

_____ TUESDAY

GOAL:

_____

HOW I'M FEELING:

_____
_____

HOW THE BABY IS DOING:

_____
_____

WHAT ELSE IS GOING ON:

_____
_____

_____ WEDNESDAY

GOAL:

_____

HOW I'M FEELING:

_____
_____

HOW THE BABY IS DOING:

_____
_____

WHAT ELSE IS GOING ON:

_____
_____

_____THURSDAY

GOAL:

HOW I'M FEELING:

HOW THE BABY IS DOING:

WHAT ELSE IS GOING ON:

_____ FRIDAY

GOAL:

HOW I'M FEELING:

HOW THE BABY IS DOING:

WHAT ELSE IS GOING ON:

_____ SATURDAY

_____ SUNDAY

_____ MONDAY

GOAL:

HOW I'M FEELING:

HOW THE BABY IS DOING:

WHAT ELSE IS GOING ON:

_____ TUESDAY

GOAL:

HOW I'M FEELING:

HOW THE BABY IS DOING:

WHAT ELSE IS GOING ON:

_____ WEDNESDAY

GOAL:

HOW I'M FEELING:

HOW THE BABY IS DOING:

WHAT ELSE IS GOING ON:

_____ THURSDAY

GOAL:

HOW I'M FEELING:

HOW THE BABY IS DOING:

WHAT ELSE IS GOING ON:

_____ FRIDAY

GOAL:

HOW I'M FEELING:

HOW THE BABY IS DOING:

WHAT ELSE IS GOING ON:

_____ SATURDAY

_____ SUNDAY

MONDAY

GOAL:

HOW I'M FEELING:

HOW THE BABY IS DOING:

WHAT ELSE IS GOING ON:

TUESDAY

GOAL:

HOW I'M FEELING:

HOW THE BABY IS DOING:

WHAT ELSE IS GOING ON:

WEDNESDAY

GOAL:

HOW I'M FEELING:

HOW THE BABY IS DOING:

WHAT ELSE IS GOING ON:

_____ THURSDAY

GOAL:

_____

HOW I'M FEELING:

_____

_____

HOW THE BABY IS DOING:

_____

_____

WHAT ELSE IS GOING ON:

_____

_____ FRIDAY

GOAL:

_____

HOW I'M FEELING:

_____

_____

HOW THE BABY IS DOING:

_____

_____

WHAT ELSE IS GOING ON:

_____

_____ SATURDAY

_____ SUNDAY

_____ MONDAY

GOAL:
_____
_____
HOW I'M FEELING:
_____
_____
HOW THE BABY IS DOING:
_____
_____
WHAT ELSE IS GOING ON:
_____

_____ TUESDAY

GOAL:
_____
_____
HOW I'M FEELING:
_____
_____
HOW THE BABY IS DOING:
_____
_____
WHAT ELSE IS GOING ON:
_____

_____ WEDNESDAY

GOAL:
_____
_____
HOW I'M FEELING:
_____
_____
HOW THE BABY IS DOING:
_____
_____
WHAT ELSE IS GOING ON:
_____

_____ THURSDAY

GOAL: _____

HOW I'M FEELING: _____
_____

HOW THE BABY IS DOING: _____
_____

WHAT ELSE IS GOING ON: _____

_____ FRIDAY

GOAL: _____

HOW I'M FEELING: _____
_____

HOW THE BABY IS DOING: _____
_____

WHAT ELSE IS GOING ON: _____

_____ SATURDAY

_____ SUNDAY

_____ MONDAY

GOAL:

HOW I'M FEELING:

HOW THE BABY IS DOING:

WHAT ELSE IS GOING ON:

_____ TUESDAY

GOAL:

HOW I'M FEELING:

HOW THE BABY IS DOING:

WHAT ELSE IS GOING ON:

_____ WEDNESDAY

GOAL:

HOW I'M FEELING:

HOW THE BABY IS DOING:

WHAT ELSE IS GOING ON:

_____THURSDAY

GOAL:

HOW I'M FEELING:

HOW THE BABY IS DOING:

WHAT ELSE IS GOING ON:

_____ FRIDAY

GOAL:

HOW I'M FEELING:

HOW THE BABY IS DOING:

WHAT ELSE IS GOING ON:

_____ SATURDAY

_____ SUNDAY

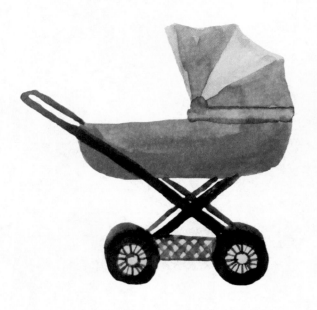

To Be Read to Your Sweet Baby on the Last Day of Nursing

Sweet child of mine. You are my heart. You are my love. Today is the last day I will nurse you. You can nurse for as long as you want, and then it will be done. No matter what, you are my love and I am here for you.

WE ARE FOREVER TOGETHER AND FOREVER APART. I LOVE YOU

_____

(name of child), and I am here for you always.

_____

_____

_____

_____

_____

_____

Dear Mothers,

Congratulations on nursing, weaning, and giving this gift of memories to yourself and your child. This is a milestone of epic proportions.

When weaning, there can be unexpected rage, sadness, and an overwhelming feeling that can be shocking and hard to navigate.

You are seen. You are loved.

_____

_____

_____

_____

_____

_____

_____

_____

_____

_____

_____

_____

MY HEART IS BROKEN AS THE HEART OUTSIDE
ME GROWS, AND SO IN TURN—IT HEALS.

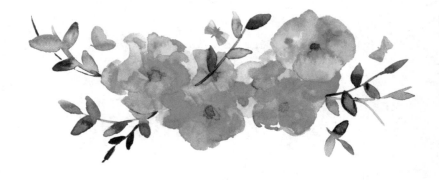

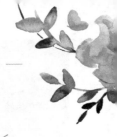

About the Author

Alisha Gaddis is an Emmy Award-winning actor, multiple Latin Grammy Award-winner, television writer, author, publisher (Little Maven Books), and international children's media star.

She is a graduate of New York University's Tisch School of the Arts and the University of Sydney, Australia. Alisha's first book *Comedic Monologues for Women that are Actually Funny*, released via Applause Books in 2014, became a bestseller. Alisha also stars in the PBS children's program that she co-created, *Lishy Lou and Lucky Too* (via The Friday Zone). Alongside her husband, Lucky Diaz, she is the cofounder and performer for the Latin Grammy Award-winning band—Lucky Diaz and the Family Jam Band. Their music has topped the charts at Sirius XM and is *People Magazine*'s #1 album of the year.

When she isn't touring the world with her and her husband's band, she splits her time between Los Angeles, CA, and Columbus, IN. Although she has many jobs, the one she loves the most is that of being a mama.

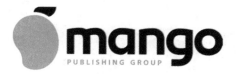

Mango Publishing, established in 2014, publishes an eclectic list of books by diverse authors—both new and established voices—on topics ranging from business, personal growth, women's empowerment, LGBTQ studies, health, and spirituality to history, popular culture, time management, decluttering, lifestyle, mental wellness, aging, and sustainable living. We were recently named 2019 and 2020's #1 fastest growing independent publisher by Publishers Weekly. Our success is driven by our main goal, which is to publish high quality books that will entertain readers as well as make a positive difference in their lives.

Our readers are our most important resource; we value your input, suggestions, and ideas. We'd love to hear from you—after all, we are publishing books for you!

Please stay in touch with us and follow us at:

Facebook: Mango Publishing
Twitter: @MangoPublishing
Instagram: @MangoPublishing
LinkedIn: Mango Publishing
Pinterest: Mango Publishing

Newsletter: mangopublishinggroup.com/newsletter

Join us on Mango's journey to reinvent publishing, one book at a time.